Pescatarian Cookbook 2021

The Most Comprehensive Cookbook for your Seafood and Vegetarian Diet Plan

Lara Dillard

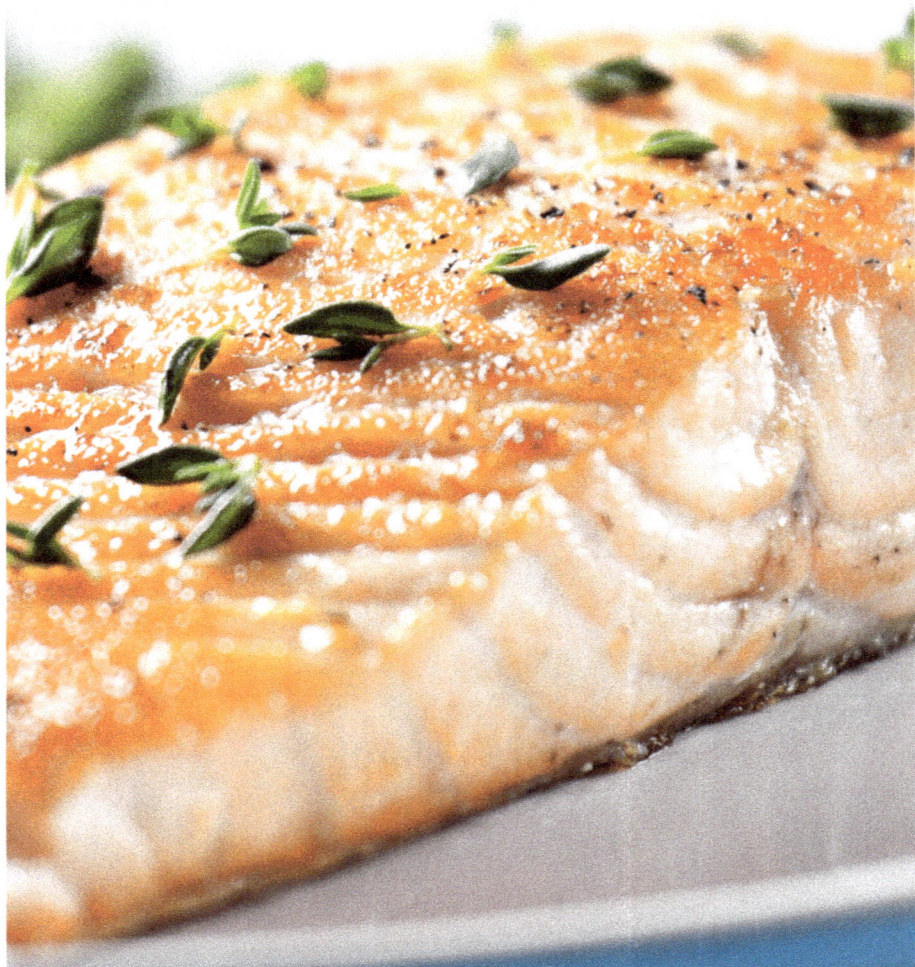

by reading this document, the reader agrees that under no circumstances is the author responsible for any losses, direct or indirect, which are incurred as a result of the use of information contained within this document, including, but not limited to, — errors, omissions, or inaccuracies.

Table of Contents

Perfect Parmesan Salmon

Preparation Time: 10 minutes

Cooking Time: 10 minutes

Serve: 4

Nutritional Value (Amount per Serving):

- Calories 294
- Fat 16 g
- Carbohydrates 3.7 g
- Sugar 1 g
- Protein 34.8 g
- Cholesterol 82 mg

Ingredients:

- 4 salmon fillets
- 1/4 cup parmesan cheese, shredded
- 1/4 tsp dried dill

- 1/2 tbsp Dijon mustard
- 4 tbsp mayonnaise
- 1 lemon juice
- Pepper
- Salt

Directions:

1. In a small bowl, mix cheese, dill, mustard, mayonnaise, lemon juice, pepper, and salt.

2. Place salmon fillets into the air fryer basket and brush with cheese mixture.

3. Cook salmon fillets at 400 F for 10 minutes.

4. Serve and enjoy.

Quick & Easy Salmon

Preparation Time: 10 minutes

Cooking Time: 8 minutes

Serve: 4

Nutritional Value (Amount per Serving):

- Calories 269
- Fat 14.5 g
- Carbohydrates 0.7 g
- Sugar 0.2 g
- Protein 34.7 g
- Cholesterol 78 mg

Ingredients:

- 4 salmon fillets
- 1/2 tsp smoked paprika
- 1 tsp garlic powder

- 1 tbsp olive oil
- Pepper
- Salt

Directions:

1. Preheat the air fryer to 400 F.

2. Brush salmon fillets with oil and sprinkle with smoked paprika, garlic powder, pepper, and salt.

3. Place salmon fillets into the air fryer basket and cook for 8 minutes.

4. Serve and enjoy.

Healthy Salmon Patties

Preparation Time: 10 minutes

Cooking Time: 8 minutes

Serve: 6

Nutritional Value (Amount per Serving):

- Calories 105
- Fat 4.8 g
- Carbohydrates 0.7 g
- Sugar 0.2 g
- Protein 14.2 g
- Cholesterol 64 mg

Ingredients:

- 1 egg
- 1 tsp paprika
- 2 green onions, minced

- 2 tbsp fresh coriander, chopped
- 14 oz can salmon, drain & mince
- Pepper
- Salt

Directions:

1. Preheat the air fryer to 360 F.

2. Add all ingredients into the bowl and mix until well combined.

3. Spray air fryer basket with cooking spray.

4. Make the equal shape of patties from the mixture and place into the air fryer basket and cook for 8 minutes.

5. Serve and enjoy.

Flavorful Salmon Fillets

Preparation Time: 10 minutes

Cooking Time: 10 minutes

Serve: 2

Nutritional Value (Amount per Serving):

- Calories 366
- Fat 25.4 g
- Carbohydrates 1.5 g
- Sugar 0.6 g
- Protein 35 g
- Cholesterol 78 mg

Ingredients:

- 2 salmon fillets, boneless
- 1/2 tsp garlic powder
- 1/2 tsp ground cumin

- 1/2 tsp chili powder
- 2 tbsp fresh lemon juice
- 2 tbsp olive oil
- Pepper
- Salt

Directions:

1. In a small bowl, mix oil, lemon juice, chili powder, ground cumin, garlic powder, pepper, and salt.

2. Brush salmon fillets with oil mixture and place into the air fryer basket and cook at 400 F for 10 minutes.

3. Serve and enjoy.

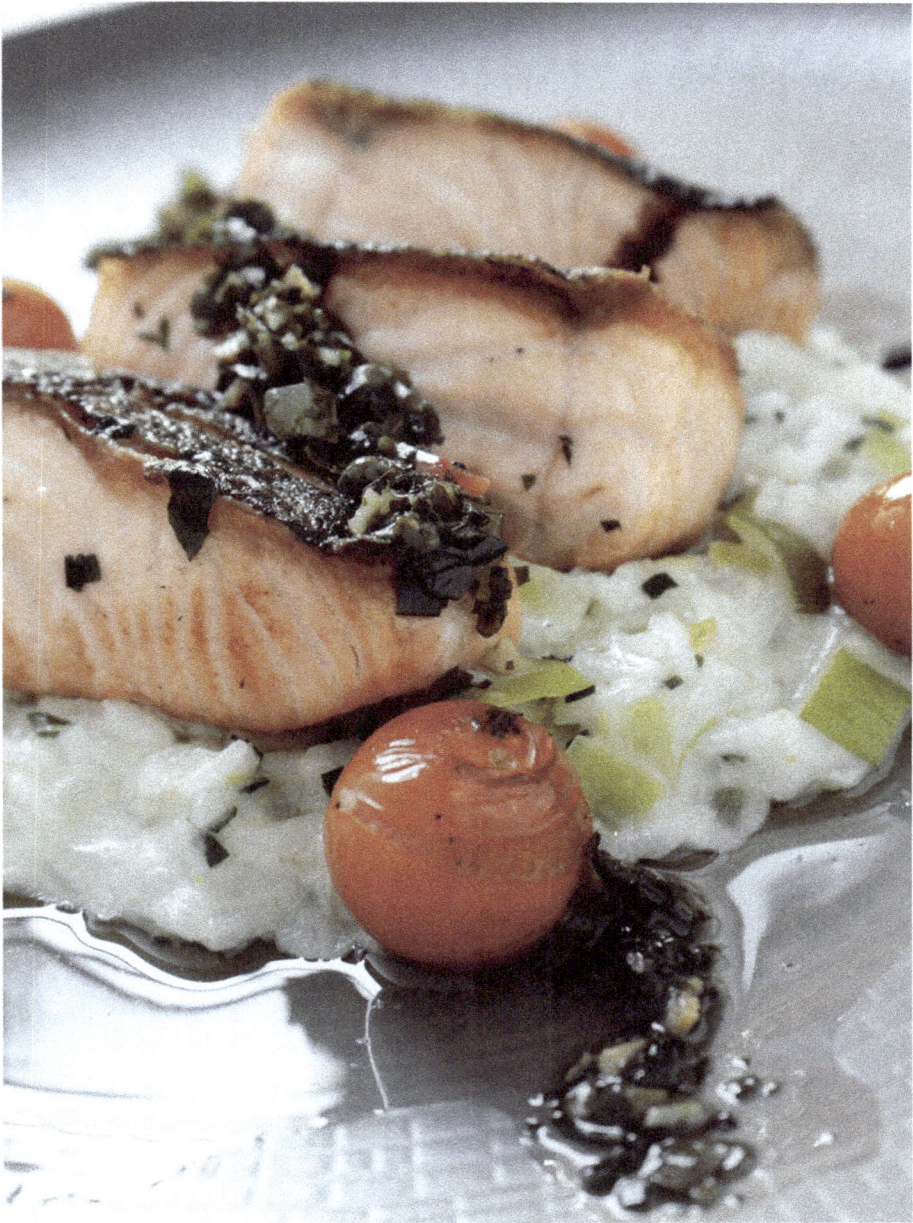

Basil Cheese Salmon

Preparation Time: 10 minutes

Cooking Time: 7 minutes

Serve: 4

Nutritional Value (Amount per Serving):

- Calories 414
- Fat 22.4 g
- Carbohydrates 1.8 g
- Sugar 0.5 g
- Protein 46.6 g
- Cholesterol 110 mg

Ingredients:

- 4 salmon fillets
- 1/4 cup parmesan cheese, grated
- 5 fresh basil leaves, minced

- 2 tbsp mayonnaise
- 1/2 lemon juice
- Pepper
- Salt

Directions:

1. Preheat the air fryer to 400 F.

2. Brush salmon fillets with lemon juice and season with pepper and salt.

3. In a small bowl, mix mayonnaise, basil, and cheese.

4. Spray air fryer basket with cooking spray.

5. Place salmon fillets into the air fryer basket and brush with mayonnaise mixture and cook for 7 minutes.

6. Serve and enjoy.

Sriracha Salmon

Preparation Time: 10 minutes

Cooking Time: 12 minutes

Serve: 4

Ingredients:

- 1 lb salmon fillets
- 1 tbsp soy sauce
- 1/2 cup honey
- 4 tbsp sriracha

Nutritional Value (Amount per Serving):

- Calories 296
- Fat 7 g
- Carbohydrates 38.2 g
- Sugar 34.9 g
- Protein 22.4 g

- Cholesterol 50 mg

Directions:

1. In a bowl, mix soy sauce, honey, and sriracha. Add fish fillets and mix well, cover and place in the refrigerator for 30 minutes.

2. Spray air fryer basket with cooking spray.

3. Place marinated salmon fillets into the air fryer basket and cook at 400 F for 12 minutes.

4. Serve and enjoy.

Garlic Brown Sugar Salmon

Preparation Time: 10 minutes

Cooking Time: 10 minutes

Serve: 4

Ingredients:

- 1 lb salmon fillets
- 3/4 tsp garlic powder
- 1 tsp Italian seasoning
- 1/2 tsp smoked paprika
- 3/4 tsp chili powder
- 2 tbsp brown sugar
- Pepper
- Salt

Nutritional Value (Amount per Serving):

- Calories 175

- Fat 7.5 g
- Carbohydrates 5.4 g
- Sugar 4.7 g
- Protein 22.2 g
- Cholesterol 51 mg

Directions:

1. In a small bowl, mix garlic powder, Italian seasoning, paprika, chili powder, brown sugar, pepper, and salt and rub over salmon fillets.
2. Spray air fryer basket with cooking spray.
3. Place salmon fillets into the air fryer basket and cook at 400 F for 10 minutes.
4. Serve and enjoy.

Blackened Salmon

Preparation Time: 10 minutes

Cooking Time: 7 minutes

Serve: 4

Nutritional Value (Amount per Serving):

Calories 274

Fat 14.8 g

Carbohydrates 1.7 g

Sugar 0.3 g

Protein 34.9 g

Cholesterol 78 mg

Ingredients:

- 4 salmon fillets

- 3/4 tsp dried thyme
- 3/4 tsp dried oregano
- 1/2 tsp garlic powder
- 1/2 tsp cayenne
- 1 tbsp sweet paprika
- 1 tbsp olive oil
- Pepper
- Salt

Directions:

1. Preheat the air fryer to 400 F.

2. In a small bowl, mix thyme, oregano, garlic powder, cayenne, paprika, pepper, and salt.

3. Brush salmon fillets with oil and coat with spice and herb mixture.

4. Place salmon fillets into the air fryer basket and cook for 7 minutes.

5. Serve and enjoy.

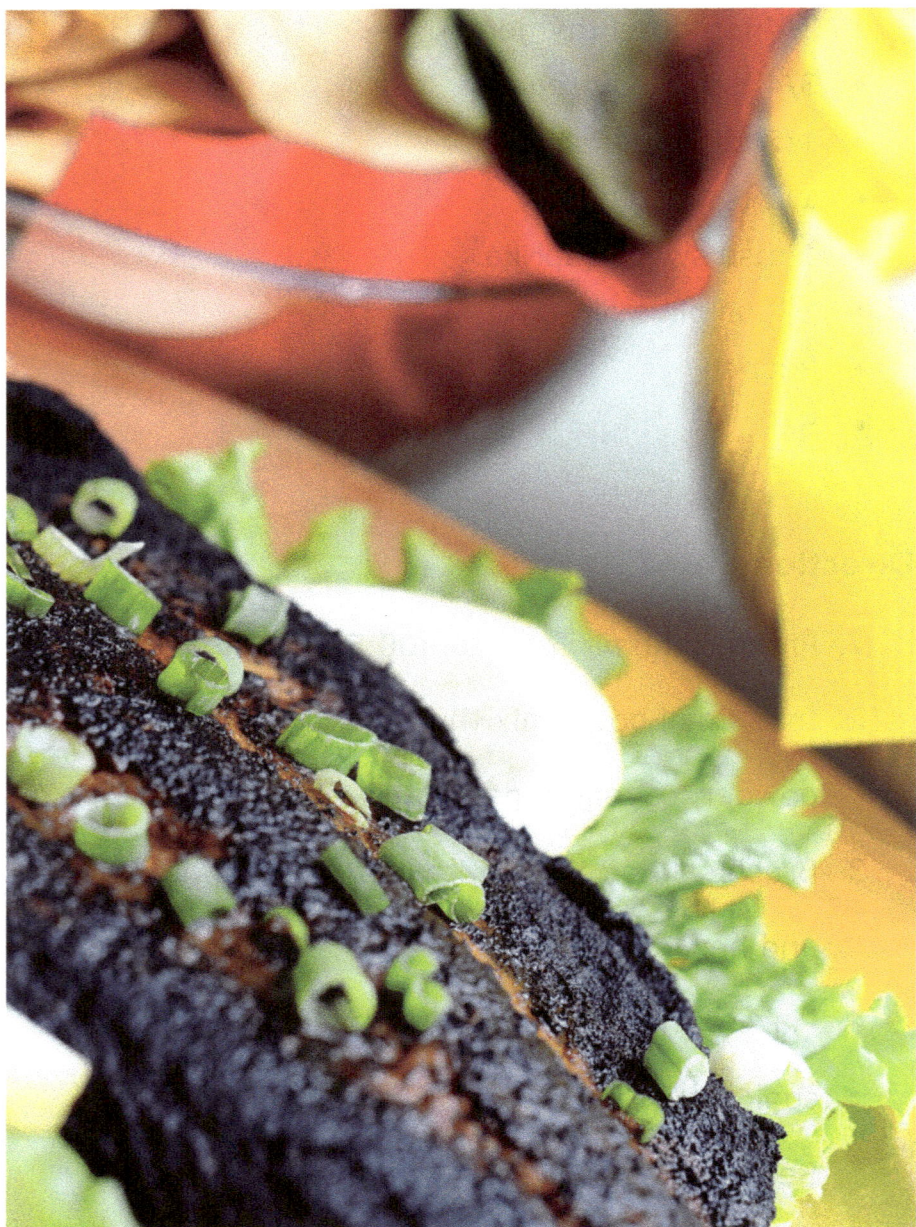

Honey Mustard Salmon

Preparation Time: 10 minutes

Cooking Time: 10 minutes

Serve: 2

Nutritional Value (Amount per Serving):

- Calories 296
- Fat 13.8 g
- Carbohydrates 9.7 g
- Sugar 8.8 g
- Protein 35.1 g
- Cholesterol 78 mg

Ingredients:

- 2 salmon fillets
- 1 tsp paprika
- 1 tsp olive oil

- 1 tbsp Dijon mustard
- 1 tbsp honey
- Pepper
- Salt

Directions:

1. Preheat the air fryer to 400 F.

2. In a small bowl, mix honey, mustard, oil, paprika, pepper, and salt.

3. Brush salmon fillets with honey mixture and place into the air fryer basket and cook for 10 minutes.

4. Serve and enjoy.

Chili Sauce Salmon

Preparation Time: 10 minutes

Cooking Time: 15 minutes

Serve: 2

Nutritional Value (Amount per Serving):

- Calories 541
- Fat 33.6 g
- Carbohydrates 16.3 g
- Sugar 3.8 g
- Protein 44.5 g
- Cholesterol 115 mg

Ingredients:

- 1 lb salmon fillets
- 1 1/2 tbsp sriracha
- 1/3 cup Thai chili sauce

- 1/2 cup mayonnaise
- Pepper
- Salt

Directions:

1. In a small bowl, mix sriracha, chili sauce, mayonnaise, pepper, and salt.

2. Brush salmon fillets with sriracha mixture and place into the air fryer basket and cook at 400 F for 13-15 minutes.

3. Serve and enjoy.

Easy Cod Fillet

Preparation Time: 10 minutes

Cooking Time: 10 minutes

Serve: 1

Nutritional Value (Amount per Serving):

- Calories 72
- Fat 0.4 g
- Carbohydrates 1 g
- Sugar 0.3 g
- Protein 16.9 g
- Cholesterol 27 mg

Ingredients:

- 3 oz cod fillet
- 1/8 tsp garlic powder
- 1 lemon slice

- Pepper
- Salt

Directions:

1. Season cod fillet with garlic powder, pepper, and salt.

2. Place cod fillet into the air fryer basket and top with a lemon slice.

3. Cook cod fillet at 375 F for 10 minutes.

4. Serve and enjoy.

Lemon Dill Cod

Preparation Time: 10 minutes

Cooking Time: 10 minutes

Serve: 4

Nutritional Value (Amount per Serving):

Calories 204

Fat 12.3 g

Carbohydrates 1.4 g

Sugar 0.2 g

Protein 21.2 g

Cholesterol 73 mg

Ingredients:

- 4 cod fillets

- 1 tsp dried dill
- 2 tbsp lemon juice
- 1 1/2 tbsp garlic, minced
- 1/4 cup butter, melted
- Pepper
- Salt

Directions:

1. Preheat the air fryer to 370 F.

2. In a bowl, mix butter, garlic, lemon juice, dill, pepper, and salt. Add cod fillets and coat well.

3. Place fish fillets into the air fryer basket and cook for 10 minutes.

4. Serve and enjoy.

Quick Chili Lime Cod

Preparation Time: 10 minutes

Cooking Time: 10 minutes

Serve: 2

Nutritional Value (Amount per Serving):

Calories 159

Fat 8.3 g

Carbohydrates 1.7 g

Sugar 0.3 g

Protein 20.4 g

Cholesterol 40 mg

Ingredients:

- 2 cod fillets

- 1 tbsp olive oil
- 1/4 tsp ground cumin
- 1/2 tsp garlic powder
- 1/2 tsp chili powder
- 1/2 tsp dried oregano
- 1 tsp dried parsley
- 3/4 tsp smoked paprika
- 1 lime zest, grated
- Salt

Directions:

1. Add oil, cumin, garlic powder, chili powder, oregano, parsley, paprika, and salt into the zip-lock bag and mix well.

2. Add cod fillets into the zip-lock bag, seal bag, and place in the refrigerator for 30 minutes.

3. Preheat the air fryer to 380 F.

4. Place marinated fish fillets into the air fryer basket and cook for 10 minutes.

5. Serve and enjoy.

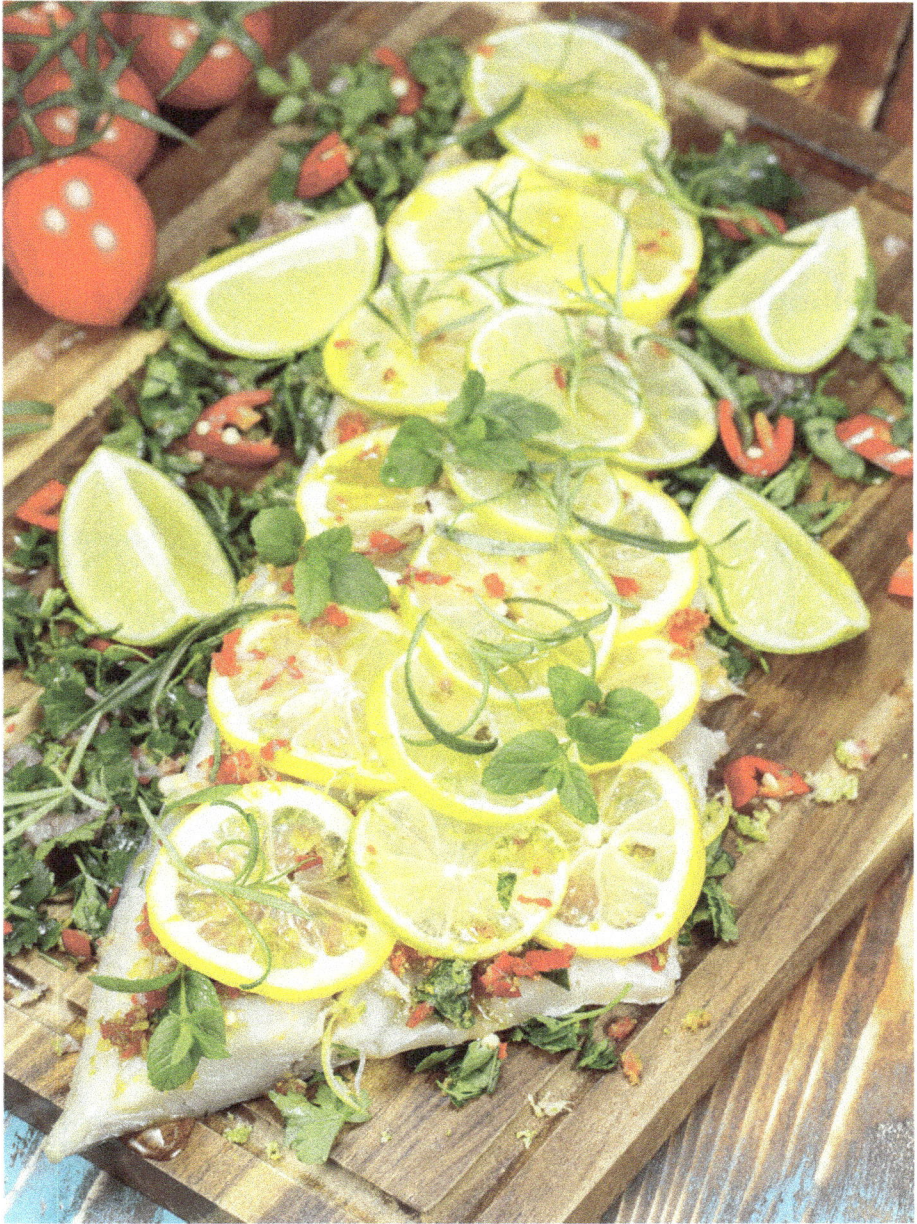

Parmesan Cod Fillets

Preparation Time: 10 minutes

Cooking Time: 7 minutes

Serve: 2

Nutritional Value (Amount per Serving):

Calories 619

Fat 34.6 g

Carbohydrates 19.5 g

Sugar 1.7 g

Protein 47.6 g

Cholesterol 115 mg

Ingredients:

- 2 cod fillets

- 1/4 cup parmesan cheese, grated
- 1/2 cup whole-wheat breadcrumbs
- 1/4 tsp Italian seasoning
- 2 tbsp olive oil
- Pepper
- Salt

Directions:

1. In a shallow dish, mix parmesan cheese, breadcrumbs, Italian seasoning, pepper, and salt.
2. Brush fish fillets with oil and coat with cheese mixture.
3. Place fish fillets into the air fryer basket and cook at 390 F for 7 minutes.
4. Serve and enjoy.

Miso Sea Bass Fillets

Preparation Time: 10 minutes

Cooking Time: 20 minutes

Serve: 2

Nutritional Value (Amount per Serving)

- Calories 408
- Fat 11.7 g
- Carbohydrates 50.8 g
- Sugar 40.7 g
- Protein 28 g
- Cholesterol 54 mg

Ingredients:

- 2 sea bass fillets
- 1/2 tsp ginger garlic paste
- 2 tbsp mirin
- 4 tbsp honey

- 1 tbsp vinegar
- 4 tbsp miso paste
- 1 tbsp olive oil
- Pepper
- Salt

Directions:

1. Preheat the air fryer to 375 F.

2. Spray fish fillets with cooking spray and season with pepper and salt.

3. Place fish fillets into the air fryer basket and cook for 15 minutes.

4. Meanwhile, heat oil in a pan over medium heat. Add miso paste, vinegar, honey, mirin, and ginger garlic paste and stir to combine.

5. Remove pan from heat. Brush fish fillets with a miso glaze.

6. Serve and enjoy.

Curried Cod Fillets

Preparation Time: 10 minutes

Cooking Time: 10 minutes

Serve: 2

Nutritional Value (Amount per Serving):

- Calories 181
- Fat 9.4 g
- Carbohydrates 4.4 g
- Sugar 3.5 g
- Protein 20.2 g
- Cholesterol 60 mg

Ingredients:

- 2 cod fillets
- 1/8 tsp smoked paprika
- 1/8 tsp curry powder

- 1/8 tsp garlic powder
- 1/2 tsp sugar
- 1/4 cup Italian dressing
- Pepper
- Salt

Directions:

1. Add fish fillets and remaining ingredients into the bowl and mix well. Cover and place in the refrigerator for 15 minutes.
2. Preheat the air fryer to 370 F.
3. Spray air fryer basket with cooking spray.
4. Place fish fillets into the air fryer basket and cook for 10 minutes.
5. Serve and enjoy.

Garlic Lemon Tilapia

Preparation Time: 10 minutes

Cooking Time: 10 minutes

Serve: 2

Nutritional Value (Amount per Serving):

- Calories 97
- Fat 1.1 g
- Carbohydrates 0.9 g
- Sugar 0.2 g
- Protein 21.2 g
- Cholesterol 55 mg

Ingredients:

- 2 tilapia fillets
- 1/2 tsp lemon pepper seasoning
- 1/2 tsp garlic powder

- Pepper
- Salt

Directions:

1. Preheat the air fryer to 360 F.

2. Spray fish fillets with cooking spray.

3. Season fish fillets with lemon pepper seasoning, garlic powder, pepper, and salt.

4. Place fish fillets into the air fryer basket and cook for 10 minutes.

5. Serve and enjoy.

Super Healthy Tilapia

Preparation Time: 10 minutes

Cooking Time: 10 minutes

Serve: 2

Nutritional Value (Amount per Serving):

- Calories 183
- Fat 6.7 g
- Carbohydrates 0.7 g
- Sugar 0.2 g
- Protein 32.2 g
- Cholesterol 85 mg

Ingredients:

- 2 tilapia fillets
- 1/4 tsp smoked paprika
- 1/2 tsp garlic powder

- 2 tsp olive oil
- Pepper
- Salt

Directions:

1. Preheat the air fryer to 390 F.

2. Brush fish fillets with oil and sprinkle with paprika, garlic powder, pepper, and salt.

3. Place fish fillets into the air fryer basket and cook for 10 minutes.

4. Serve and enjoy.

Flavorful Halibut

Preparation Time: 10 minutes

Cooking Time: 12 minutes

Serve: 2

Ingredients:

- 2 halibut fillets
- 1/2 tsp onion powder
- 1/2 tsp garlic powder
- 1/4 tsp chili powder
- Pepper
- Salt

Nutritional Value (Amount per Serving):

- Calories 324
- Fat 6.8 g
- Carbohydrates 1.2 g

- Sugar 0.4 g
- Protein 60.7 g
- Cholesterol 93 mg

Directions:

1. Spray fish fillets with cooking spray.

2. Season fish fillets with onion powder, garlic powder, chili powder, pepper, and salt.

3. Place fish fillets into the air fryer basket and cook for 12 minutes.

4. Serve and enjoy.

Crispy Crusted Halibut

Preparation Time: 10 minutes

Cooking Time: 10 minutes

Serve: 4

Nutritional Value (Amount per Serving):

- Calories 467
- Fat 7.6 g
- Carbohydrates 25.3 g
- Sugar 1.2 g
- Protein 64.2 g
- Cholesterol 93 mg

Ingredients:

- 4 halibut fillets
- 1/2 cup white wine
- 1/2 cup cornstarch

- 2 egg whites
- 1/2 cup whole-wheat breadcrumbs
- 1/2 cup pecan, crushed
- 1/2 tsp Italian seasoning
- Pepper
- Salt

Directions:

1. In a bowl, whisk together egg whites, cornstarch, and wine.

2. In a shallow dish, mix breadcrumbs, pecans, Italian seasoning, pepper, and salt.

3. Dredge the fish fillets into the egg mixture then coat with breadcrumb mixture.

4. Preheat the air fryer to 375 F.

5. Spray air fryer basket with cooking spray.

6. Place fish fillets into the air fryer basket and cook for 10 minutes.

7. Serve and enjoy.

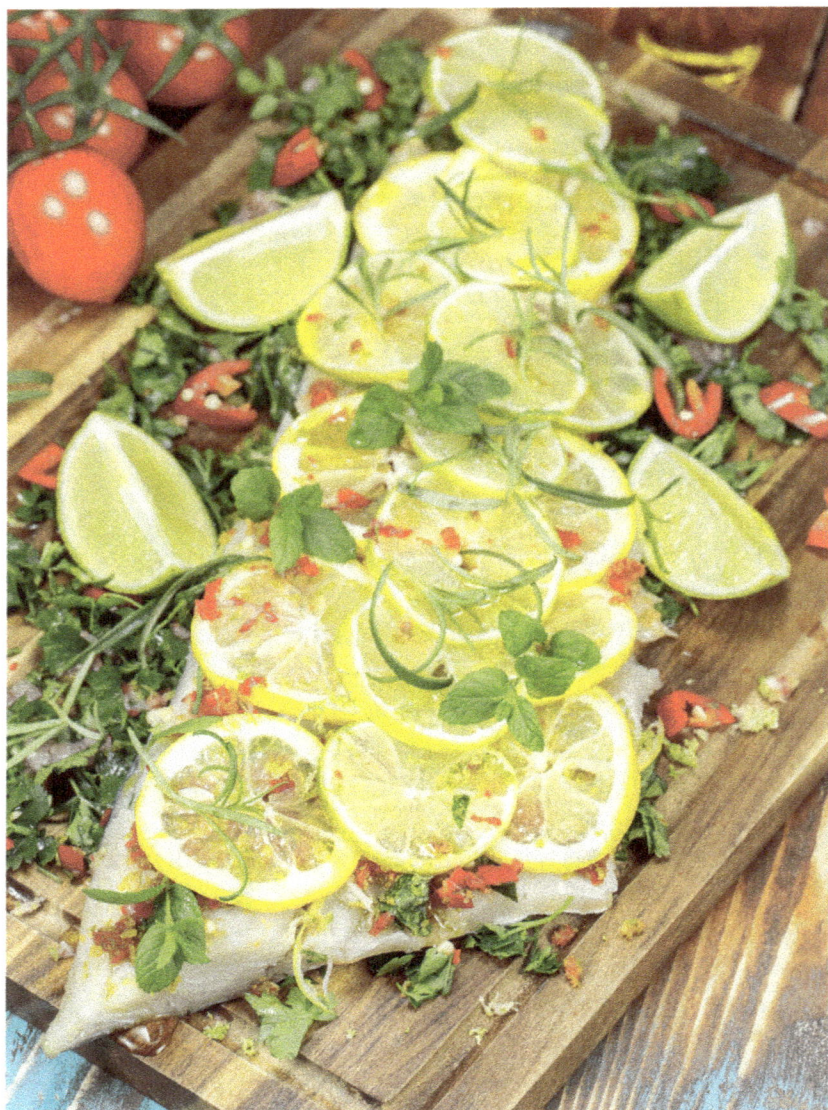

Parmesan Halibut

Preparation Time: 10 minutes

Cooking Time: 15 minutes

Serve: 2

Nutritional Value (Amount per Serving):

- Calories 380
- Fat 13.7 g
- Carbohydrates 0.4 g
- Sugar 0.1 g
- Protein 60.6 g
- Cholesterol 93 mg

Ingredients:

- 2 halibut fillets
- 1/4 tsp garlic powder
- 1 tbsp parsley, chopped

- 1/4 cup parmesan cheese, grated
- 1/2 cup whole-wheat breadcrumbs
- 1/2 lemon juice
- 1 tbsp olive oil
- Pepper
- Salt

Directions:

1. In a shallow dish, mix breadcrumbs, cheese, parsley, garlic powder, pepper, and salt.
2. In a small bowl, mix oil and lemon juice.
3. Brush fish fillets with oil mixture and coat with breadcrumb mixture.
4. Place fish fillets into the air fryer basket and cook at 400 F for 12-15 minutes.
5. Serve and enjoy.

Garlic Herb Tilapia

Preparation Time: 10 minutes

Cooking Time: 12 minutes

Serve: 4

Nutritional Value (Amount per Serving):

- Calories 130
- Fat 4.5 g
- Carbohydrates 0 g
- Sugar 0 g
- Protein 22 g
- Cholesterol 100 mg

Ingredients:

- 4 tilapia fillets
- 1 tbsp olive oil
- 1 tbsp garlic herb seasoning

Directions:

1. Preheat the air fryer to 400 F.

2. Brush fish fillets with oil and sprinkle with seasoning.

3. Place fish fillets into the air fryer basket and cook for 12 minutes.

4. Serve and enjoy.

Crispy Catfish Fillets

Preparation Time: 10 minutes

Cooking Time: 20 minutes

Serve: 4

Nutritional Value (Amount per Serving):

- Calories 326
- Fat 13.2 g
- Carbohydrates 23.5 g
- Sugar 0.2 g
- Protein 27.4 g
- Cholesterol 75 mg

Ingredients:

- 4 catfish fillets
- 3 tsp Cajun seasoning
- 1 cup cornmeal
- Pepper
- Salt

Directions:

1. In a shallow dish, mix cornmeal, pepper, Cajun seasoning, and salt.

2. Coat fish fillets with cornmeal mixture and place into the air fryer basket and cook at 390 F for 15 minutes.

3. Turn temperature to 400 F and cook fish fillets for 5 minutes more.

4. Serve and enjoy.

Simple & Tasty Tilapia

Preparation Time: 10 minutes

Cooking Time: 5 minutes

Serve: 4

Nutritional Value (Amount per Serving):

- Calories 266
- Fat 13.1 g
- Carbohydrates 23.1 g
- Sugar 1.1 g
- Protein 13.4 g
- Cholesterol 66 mg

Ingredients:

- 1 egg, lightly beaten
- 1 tbsp old bay seasoning
- 1 cup whole-wheat breadcrumbs

- 4 tilapia fish fillets

Directions:

1. Preheat the air fryer to 400 F.

2. In a small dish, add egg and whisk well.

3. In a shallow dish, mix breadcrumbs and seasoning.

4. Dip fish fillets in egg then coat with breadcrumb mixture.

5. Place fish fillets into the air fryer basket and cook for 5 minutes.

6. Serve and enjoy.

Juicy & Tender Tilapia

Preparation Time: 10 minutes

Cooking Time: 10 minutes

Serve: 2

Ingredients:

- 2 tilapia fillets
- 1 tsp garlic, minced
- 2 tsp parsley, chopped
- 2 tsp chives, chopped
- 2 tsp olive oil
- Pepper
- Salt

Nutritional Value (Amount per Serving):

- Calories 143
- Fat 5.7 g

- Carbohydrates 0.6 g
- Sugar 0 g
- Protein 22.2 g
- Cholesterol 100 mg

Directions:

1. Preheat the air fryer to 400 F.

2. In a small bowl, mix oil, chives, parsley, garlic, pepper, and salt.

3. Brush fish fillets with oil mixture and place into the air fryer basket and cook for 10 minutes.

4. Serve and enjoy.

Simple Mahi Mahi

Preparation Time: 10 minutes

Cooking Time: 12 minutes

Serve: 4

Nutritional Value (Amount per Serving):

- Calories 361
- Fat 30.7 g
- Carbohydrates 0 g
- Sugar 0 g
- Protein 21.3 g
- Cholesterol 121 mg
- **Ingredients:**
- 4 mahi-mahi fillets
- 2/3 cup butter
- Pepper
- Salt

Directions:

1. Preheat the air fryer to 350 F.

2. Season Mahi-mahi fillets with pepper and salt.

3. Place fish fillets into the air fryer basket and cook for 12 minutes.

4. Add butter into the pan and melt over medium heat.

5. Pour melted butter over fish fillets and serve.

Pesto Mahi Mahi

Preparation Time: 10 minutes

Cooking Time: 15 minutes

Serve: 2

Nutritional Value (Amount per Serving):

- Calories 92
- Fat 0.1 g
- Carbohydrates 0.3 g
- Sugar 0 g
- Protein 21.3 g
- Cholesterol 40 mg

Ingredients:

- 2 mahi-mahi fillets
- 3/4 cup basil pesto
- Pepper

- Salt

Directions:

1. Preheat the air fryer to 300 F.
2. Season fish fillets with pepper and salt.
3. Place fish fillets into the air fryer basket. Top fish with basil pesto and cook for 12-15 minutes.
4. Serve and enjoy.

Easy Lemon Dill Fish Fillets

Preparation Time: 10 minutes

Cooking Time: 14 minutes

Serve: 2

Nutritional Value (Amount per Serving):

- Calories 156
- Fat 7.1 g
- Carbohydrates 1.1 g
- Sugar 0.2 g
- Protein 21.4 g
- Cholesterol 40 mg

Ingredients:

- 2 mahi-mahi fillets
- 1 tbsp dill, chopped
- 2 lemon sliced

- 1 tbsp olive oil
- 1 tbsp lemon juice
- Pepper
- Salt

Directions:

1. In a small bowl, mix olive oil and lemon juice.
2. Season fish fillets with pepper and salt and brush with oil mixture.
3. Place fish fillets into the air fryer basket and top with dill and lemon slices and cook at 400 F for 12-14 minutes.
4. Serve and enjoy.

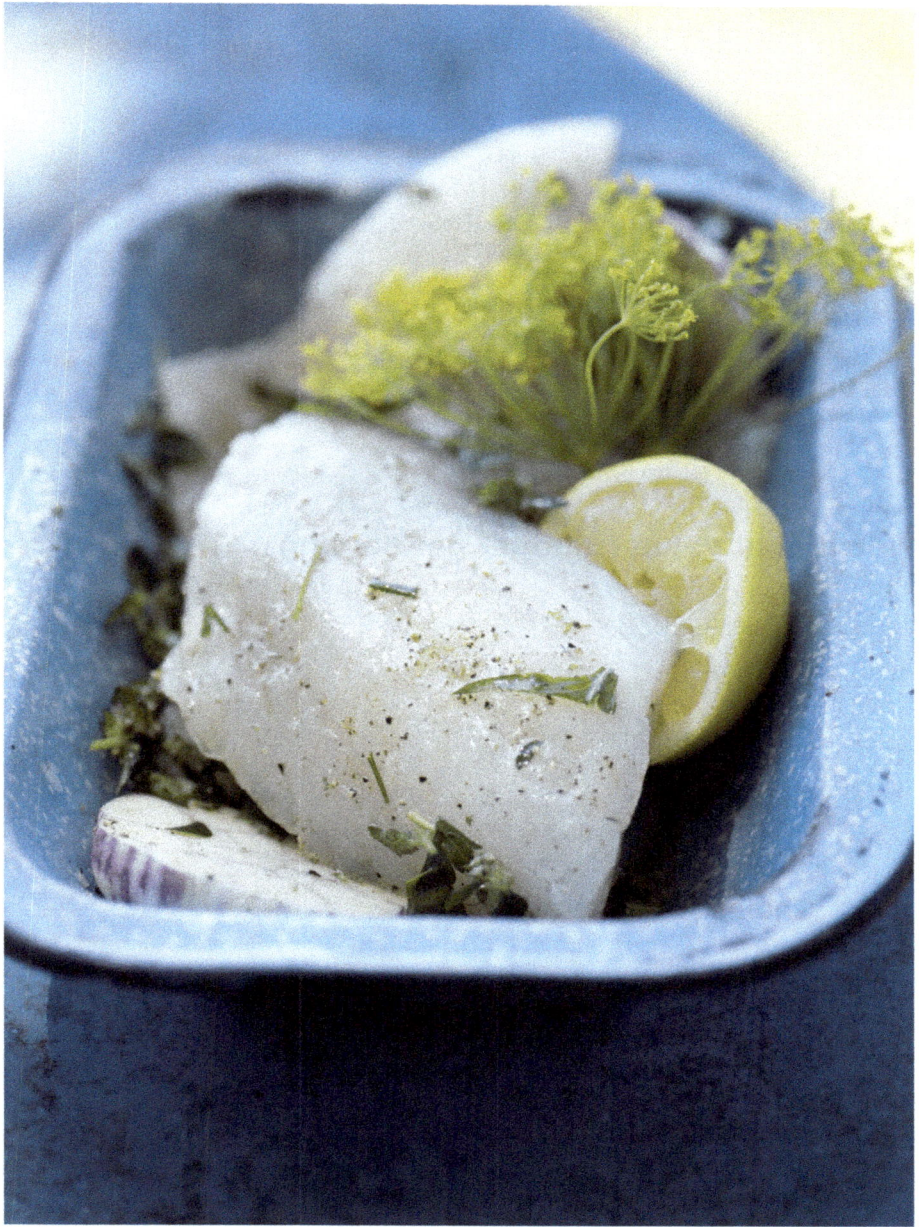

Delicious Tuna Patties

Preparation Time: 10 minutes

Cooking Time: 10 minutes

Serve: 5

Nutritional Value (Amount per Serving):

- Calories 128
- Fat 2.5 g
- Carbohydrates 0.9 g
- Sugar 0.5 g
- Protein 24.1 g
- Cholesterol 91 mg

Ingredients:

- 2 eggs, lightly beaten
- 15 oz can tuna, drained
- 1/2 tsp dried herbs
- 1/2 tsp garlic powder
- 2 tbsp onion, minced

- 1 celery stalk, chopped
- 3 tbsp parmesan cheese, grated
- 1/2 cup whole-wheat breadcrumbs
- 1 tbsp lemon juice
- 1 lemon zest
- Pepper
- Salt

Directions:

1. Add all ingredients into the bowl and mix until well combined.
2. Make equal shape of patties from mixture and place onto the parchment-lined baking sheet. Place patties in the refrigerator for 1 hour.
3. Spray air fryer basket with cooking spray.
4. Place patties into the air fryer basket and cook at 360 F for 10 minutes. Flip patties halfway through.
5. Serve and enjoy.

Cheesy Tuna Patties

Preparation Time: 10 minutes

Cooking Time: 10 minutes

Serve: 4

Nutritional Value (Amount per Serving):

- Calories 167
- Fat 8.4 g
- Carbohydrates 6.2 g
- Sugar 0.9 g
- Protein 16.3 g
- Cholesterol 65 mg

Ingredients:

- 1 egg
    - o oz tuna, drained
- 1/2 tsp onion powder

- 1/2 tsp garlic powder
- 1 tsp paprika
- 2 tbsp hot sauce
- 1 oz cheddar cheese, shredded
- 1 oz parmesan cheese, shredded
- 1/4 cup breadcrumbs
- Pepper
- Salt

Directions:

1. Add all ingredients into the bowl and mix until well combined.
2. Spray air fryer basket with cooking spray.
3. Make patties from the mixture and place into the air fryer basket and cook at 400 F for 10 minutes.
4. Serve and enjoy.

Tasty Tuna Steaks

Preparation Time: 10 minutes

Cooking Time: 10 minutes

Serve: 2

Nutritional Value (Amount per Serving):

- Calories 683
- Fat 46.4 g
- Carbohydrates 4.6 g
- Sugar 1.1 g
- Protein 61.2 g
- Cholesterol 70 mg

Ingredients:

- 1 lb tuna
- 1 tbsp garlic, minced
- 4 tbsp olive oil

- 1 tbsp garlic powder
- 1/2 tsp thyme
- Pepper
- Salt

Directions:

1. In a bowl, mix oil, garlic, garlic powder, thyme, pepper, and salt. Add tuna steaks and mix well and place in the refrigerator for 15 minutes.
2. Place tuna steaks into the air fryer basket and cook at 400 F for 10 minutes.
3. Serve and enjoy.

Flavorful Tuna Patties

Preparation Time: 10 minutes

Cooking Time: 10 minutes

Serve: 8

Nutritional Value (Amount per Serving):

- Calories 88
- Fat 3.6 g
- Carbohydrates 2.2 g
- Sugar 0.8 g
- Protein 11.3 g
- Cholesterol 57 mg

Ingredients:

- 2 eggs
- 10 oz can tuna, chopped
- 2 tbsp mayonnaise

- 1/2 tsp garlic powder
- 1/4 cup fresh mint, chopped
- 1/4 cup feta cheese, crumbled
- 1/2 onion, chopped
- Pepper
- Salt

Directions:

1. Add all ingredients into the bowl and mix until well combined.
2. spray air fryer basket with cooking spray.
3. Make patties from the mixture and place into the air fryer basket and cook at 400 F for 10 minutes.
4. Serve and enjoy.

BBQ Salmon

Preparation Time: 10 minutes

Cooking Time: 25 minutes

Serve: 4

Nutritional Value (Amount per Serving):

- Calories 323
- Fat 11.2 g
- Carbohydrates 22 g
- Sugar 20.3 g
- Protein 35.8 g
- Cholesterol 78 mg

Ingredients:

- 4 salmon fillets

For sauce:

- 2 tsp soy sauce
- 3 tbsp balsamic vinegar
- 3 tbsp brown sugar
- 1 cup tomato ketchup
- Pepper
- Salt

Directions:

1. Add all sauce ingredients into the small saucepan and bring to boil over medium heat. Turn heat to low and simmer for 15 minutes.
2. Spray salmon fillets with cooking spray and season with pepper and salt.
3. Place salmon fillets into the air fryer basket and cook at 380 for 5 minutes.
4. Brush salmon fillets with BBQ sauce and cook for 5 minutes more.
5. Serve and enjoy.

Crispy Coconut Shrimp

Preparation Time: 10 minutes

Cooking Time: 5 minutes

Serve: 4

Nutritional Value (Amount per Serving):

- Calories 184
- Fat 6.5 g
- Carbohydrates 19.1 g
- Sugar 1.3 g

- Protein 11.9 g
- Cholesterol 140 mg

Ingredients:

- 2 eggs, lightly beaten
- 20 large shrimp, peeled

- 1/4 cup whole-wheat breadcrumbs
- 1/2 cup shredded coconut
- 1/4 tsp garlic powder
- 1/2 cup all-purpose flour
- Pepper
- Salt

Directions:

1. in a small bowl, add eggs and whisk well.
2. In a shallow dish, mix breadcrumbs, shredded coconut, garlic powder, flour, pepper, and salt.
3. Preheat the air fryer to 400 F.
4. Dip shrimp in egg then coat with breadcrumb mixture.
5. Spray air fryer basket with cooking spray.
6. Place shrimp into the air fryer basket and cook for 5 minutes.
7. Serve and enjoy.

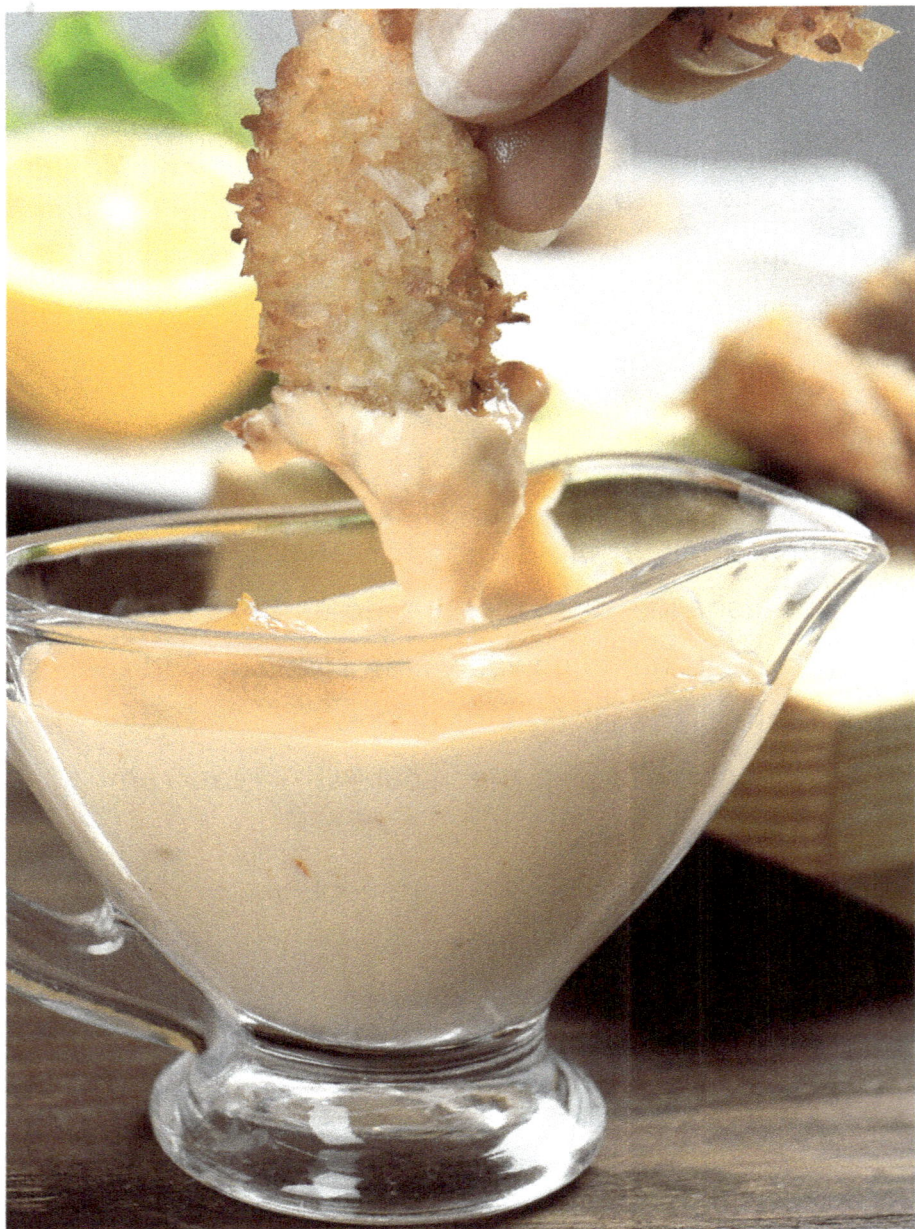

Tasty Shrimp Fajitas

Preparation Time: 10 minutes

Cooking Time: 9 minutes

Serve: 4

Nutritional Value (Amount per Serving):

- Calories 206
- Fat 5.7 g
- Carbohydrates 11.3 g
- Sugar 5.2 g
- Protein 26.9 g
- Cholesterol 239 mg

Ingredients:

- 1 lb shrimp, thawed
- 3/4 tbsp Fajita seasoning
- 1 tbsp olive oil

- 1 small onion, sliced
- 3 small bell peppers, sliced
- Pepper
- Salt

Directions:

1. Preheat the air fryer to 375 F.
2. Add shrimp and remaining ingredients into the bowl and toss well.
3. Add shrimp mixture into the air fryer basket and cook for 9 minutes. Stir halfway through.
4. Serve and enjoy.

Garlic Honey Shrimp

Preparation Time: 10 minutes

Cooking Time: 10 minutes

Serve: 6

Nutritional Value (Amount per Serving):

- Calories 229
- Fat 1.5 g
- Carbohydrates 35.1 g
- Sugar 24.7 g
- Protein 19.8 g
- Cholesterol 159 mg

Ingredients:

- 16 oz shrimp, peeled & deveined
- 16 oz mixed vegetables
- 2 tbsp cornstarch

- 1 tsp ginger garlic paste
- 2 tbsp ketchup
- 1/2 cup soy sauce
- 1/2 cup honey

Directions:

1. Add soy sauce, ketchup, ginger garlic paste, and honey into the small saucepan and cook over medium heat until warm.
2. Add cornstarch and stir constantly until thickened.
3. Remove saucepan from heat. Pour sauce over shrimp and vegetables and toss well.
4. Preheat the air fryer to 350 F.
5. Spray air fryer basket with cooking spray.
6. Add shrimp and vegetables into the air fryer basket and cook for 10 minutes.
7. Serve and enjoy.

Delicious Fish Bites

Preparation Time: 10 minutes

Cooking Time: 10 minutes

Serve: 4

Nutritional Value (Amount per Serving):

- Calories 234
- Fat 2 g
- Carbohydrates 37.7 g
- Sugar 0.2 g
- Protein 16.4 g
- Cholesterol 61 mg

Ingredients:

- 1 egg, lightly beaten
- 1 lb cod fillets, cut into 1-inch strips
- 1/2 tsp lemon pepper seasoning

- 1/2 tsp smoked paprika
- 1/2 cup whole-wheat breadcrumbs
- 1/2 cup all-purpose flour
- Pepper
- Salt

Directions:

1. In a small bowl, add egg and whisk well.
2. In a separate bowl, mix flour, pepper, and salt.
3. In a shallow dish, mix breadcrumbs, paprika, and lemon pepper seasoning.
4. Coat fish strips with flour then dip in egg and finally coat with breadcrumb mixture.
5. Preheat the air fryer to 400 F.
6. Spray air fryer basket with cooking spray.
7. Place coated fish strips into the air fryer basket and cook for 10 minutes. Turn fish strips halfway through.
8. Serve and enjoy.

Garlic Cheese Shrimp

Preparation Time: 10 minutes

Cooking Time: 8 minutes

Serve: 6

Nutritional Value (Amount per Serving):

- Calories 223
- Fat 7.3 g
- Carbohydrates 3.1 g
- Sugar 0.1 g
- Protein 34.6 g
- Cholesterol 318 mg

Ingredients:

- 2 lbs cooked shrimp, peeled & deveined
- 2 tbsp olive oil
- 3/4 tsp onion powder

- 1 tsp basil
- 1/2 tsp oregano
- 2/3 cup parmesan cheese, grated
- 1 tbsp garlic, minced
- Pepper
- Salt

Directions:

1. Add shrimp and remaining ingredients into the bowl and toss until well coated.
2. Add shrimp into the air fryer basket and cook at 350 F for 8 minutes.
3. Serve and enjoy.

Crispy Shrimp Popcorn

Preparation Time: 10 minutes

Cooking Time: 5 minutes

Serve: 4

Nutritional Value (Amount per Serving):

- Calories 356
- Fat 9.6 g
- Carbohydrates 27.6 g
- Sugar 0.2 g
- Protein 37.9 g
- Cholesterol 331 mg

Ingredients:

- 2 eggs, lightly beaten
- 5 oz oat flour
- 2 oz parmesan cheese, grated

- 8 oz whole-wheat breadcrumbs
- 1 lb shrimp, cooked & peeled
- Pepper
- Salt

Directions:

1. In a small bowl, add eggs and whisk well.
2. In a separate bowl, add oat flour.
3. In a shallow dish, mix breadcrumbs, cheese, pepper, and salt.
4. Coat shrimp with oat flour then dip in eggs and finally coat with breadcrumb mixture.
5. Place coated shrimp into the air fryer basket and cook at 400 F for 5 minutes.
6. Serve and enjoy.

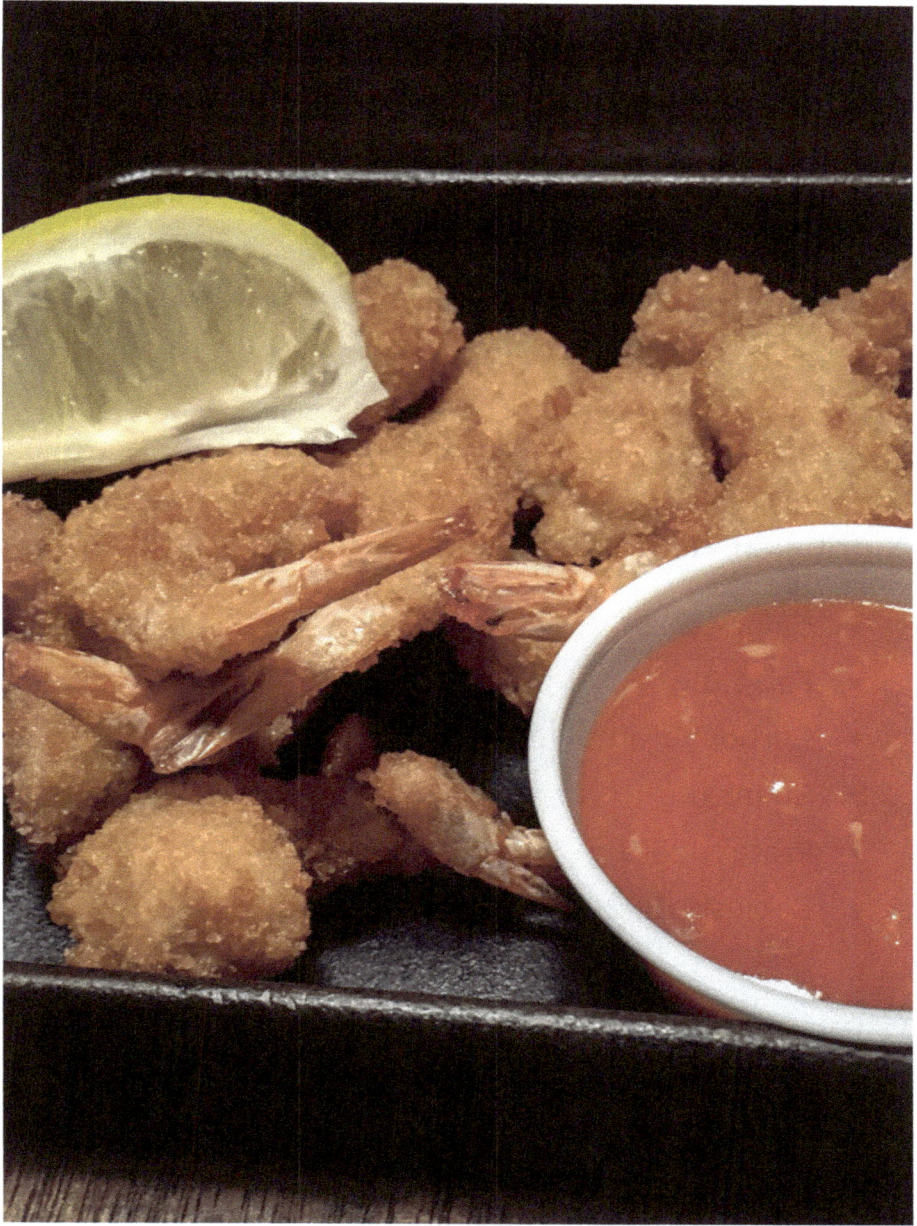

Lemon Garlic Shrimp

Preparation Time: 10 minutes

Cooking Time: 8 minutes

Serve: 4

Nutritional Value (Amount per Serving):

- Calories 161
- Fat 4.8 g
- Carbohydrates 1.9 g
- Sugar 0 g
- Protein 25.9 g
- Cholesterol 246 mg

Ingredients:

- 1 lb shrimp, peeled & deveined
- 2 tbsp parmesan cheese, grated
- 1/2 tsp garlic, minced

- 1 tsp lemon juice
- 1 tbsp butter, melted
- Salt

Directions:

1. Add shrimp and remaining ingredients into the bowl and toss well.
2. Add shrimp mixture into the air fryer basket and cook at 400 F for 8 minutes.
3. Serve and enjoy.

Shrimp Boil

Preparation Time: 10 minutes

Cooking Time: 12 minutes

Serve: 4

Nutritional Value (Amount per Serving):

- Calories 221
- Fat 14.8 g
- Carbohydrates 1.1 g
- Sugar 0.2 g
- Protein 19.4 g
- Cholesterol 131 mg

Ingredients:

- 6 oz shrimp, peeled & deveined
- 1 tbsp old bay seasoning
- 2 tbsp onion, diced

- 2 mini corn on the cobs
- 2 cups baby potatoes, boiled & halved
- 7 oz smoked sausage, sliced

Directions:

1. Add shrimp and remaining ingredients into the bowl and toss well.
2. Add shrimp mixture into the air fryer basket and cook for 12 minutes. Mix halfway through.
3. Stir well and serve.

Crispy Salt & Pepper Shrimp

Preparation Time: 10 minutes

Cooking Time: 10 minutes

Serve: 4

Nutritional Value (Amount per Serving):

- Calories 228
- Fat 9.1 g
- Carbohydrates 9.3 g
- Sugar 1 g
- Protein 26.4 g
- Cholesterol 239 mg

Ingredients:

- 1 lb shrimp
- 2 tbsp olive oil
- 3 tbsp rice flour

- 1 tsp sugar, crushed
- 2 tsp ground pepper
- Salt

Directions:

1. Add shrimp, oil, rice flour, sugar, pepper, and salt into the bowl and toss well.
2. Spray air fryer basket with cooking spray.
3. Add shrimp into the air fryer basket and cook at 325 F for 10 minutes.
4. Serve and enjoy.

Asian Shrimp

Preparation Time: 10 minutes

Cooking Time: 6 minutes

Serve: 4

Nutritional Value (Amount per Serving):

- Calories 214
- Fat 9 g
- Carbohydrates 6 g
- Sugar 3.2 g
- Protein 26.4 g
- Cholesterol 239 mg

Ingredients:

- 1 lb shrimp, peeled & deveined
- For marinade:
- 1 tbsp lemon juice

- 1 tsp garlic, minced
- 1/8 tsp cayenne
- 1 tbsp maple syrup
- 2 tbsp soy sauce
- 2 tbsp olive oil
- Pepper
- Salt

Directions:

1. Add shrimp and marinade ingredients into the bowl and mix well and place in the refrigerator for 15 minutes.
2. Spray air fryer basket with cooking spray.
3. Place shrimp into the air fryer basket and cook at 400 F for 6 minutes.
4. Serve and enjoy.

Flavorful Blackened Shrimp

Preparation Time: 10 minutes

Cooking Time: 10 minutes

Serve: 4

Nutritional Value (Amount per Serving):

- Calories 204
- Fat 9.1 g
- Carbohydrates 3.6 g
- Sugar 0.5 g
- Protein 26.2 g
- Cholesterol 239 mg

Ingredients:

- 1 lb shrimp, peeled & deveined
- 2 tsp smoked paprika
- 1/4 tsp cayenne

- 1 tsp dried oregano
- 1 tsp garlic powder
- 1 tsp onion powder
- 2 tbsp olive oil
- Pepper
- Salt

Directions:

1. Add shrimp and remaining ingredients into the bowl and toss well.
2. Preheat the air fryer to 400 F.
3. Spray air fryer basket with cooking spray.
4. Add shrimp into the air fryer basket and cook for 8-10 minutes or until cooked through.
5. Serve and enjoy.

Shrimp Dinner

Preparation Time: 10 minutes

Cooking Time: 8 minutes

Serve: 4

Nutritional Value (Amount per Serving):

- Calories 364
- Fat 21.2 g
- Carbohydrates 7.3 g
- Sugar 3.2 g
- Protein 35.6 g
- Cholesterol 275 mg

Ingredients:

- 1 lb shrimp, peeled
- 2 tbsp olive oil
- 1 bell pepper, cut into 1-inch pieces

- 1 squash, cut into slices
- 1 zucchini, cut into slices
- 6 oz sausage, sliced
- 1 tbsp Cajun seasoning
- Salt

Directions:

1. Preheat the air fryer to 400 F.
2. Add shrimp and remaining ingredients into the bowl and toss well.
3. Add shrimp mixture into the air fryer basket and cook for 8 minutes.
4. Serve and enjoy.

Shrimp with Veggie

Preparation Time: 10 minutes

Cooking Time: 15 minutes

Serve: 4

Nutritional Value (Amount per Serving):

- Calories 196
- Fat 6.6 g
- Carbohydrates 6.7 g
- Sugar 2.7 g
- Protein 26.9 g
- Cholesterol 241 mg

Ingredients:

- 1 lb shrimp, peeled & deveined
- 1/4 cup parmesan cheese, grated
- 1 tbsp Italian seasoning

- 1 tbsp garlic, minced
- 1 tbsp olive oil
- 1 bell pepper, chopped
- 1 zucchini, chopped
- Pepper
- Salt

Directions:

1. Add shrimp and remaining ingredients into the bowl and toss well.
2. Add shrimp mixture into the air fryer basket and cook at 390 F for 15 minutes. Stir halfway through.
3. Serve and enjoy.

Perfect Shrimp Skewers

Preparation Time: 10 minutes

Cooking Time: 8 minutes

Serve: 4

Nutritional Value (Amount per Serving):

- Calories 70
- Fat 1.1 g
- Carbohydrates 1.3 g
- Sugar 0 g
- Protein 13 g
- Cholesterol 119 mg

Ingredients:

- 1/2 lb shrimp, peeled & deveined
- 1 tbsp cilantro, chopped
- 1 lemon juice

- 1/2 tsp ground cumin
- 1/2 tsp smoked paprika
- 1/2 tsp garlic paste
- Salt

Directions:

1. Add shrimp and remaining ingredients into the bowl and mix well. Cover and place in the refrigerator for 15 minutes.
2. Thread shrimp onto the soaked skewers.
3. Preheat the air fryer to 350 F.
4. Place shrimp skewers into the air fryer basket and cook for 8 minutes.
5. Serve and enjoy.

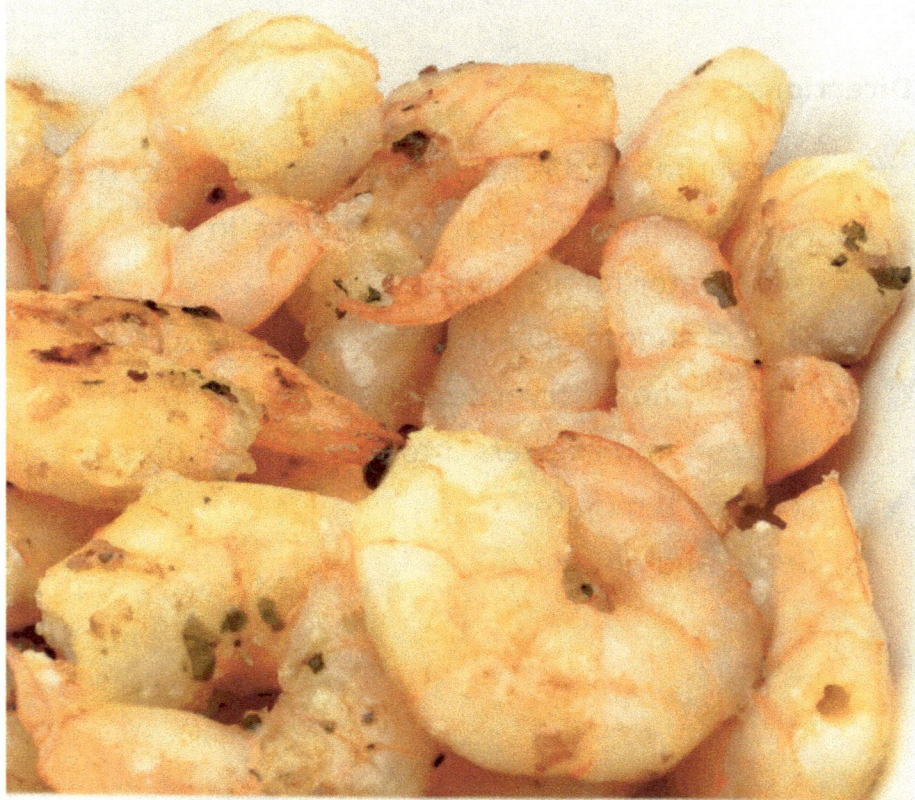

www.ingramcontent.com/pod-product-compliance
Lightning Source LLC
Chambersburg PA
CBHW070732030426
42336CB00013B/1944